Nurturing Life
Your Essential Pregnancy Guide

Table of Contents

Introduction

Welcome to the Journey of Motherhood

Congratulations! Whether this is your first pregnancy or you've been through this magical journey before, you're about to embark on one of the most life-changing experiences ever. Pregnancy is not just about creating life—it's about growth, discovery, and transformation, both for you and your baby.

This book is your companion through the highs and lows, the questions and surprises, and the joy and wonder of pregnancy. Think of it as a guide, a resource, and a friend to help you navigate the incredible path ahead.

Why This Book?

Pregnancy can feel overwhelming, with endless advice from family, friends, and the internet. It's easy to feel lost in the sea of information. That's why this book focuses on empowering you with knowledge, practical tips, and reassurance.

Whether you're wondering what foods are safe, how to prepare your body, or what labor might feel like, this book has the answers. We'll break down medical jargon, address your concerns, and share expert-backed advice, so you can feel confident and prepared every step of the way.

What You'll Find Here

This book is divided into clear, easy-to-follow sections that guide you from the very first signs of pregnancy to the moment you meet your baby—and beyond. We'll discuss:

- What to expect during each trimester.

- Practical ways to care for your body and mind.

- Preparing your home and heart for a new life.

- Handling common concerns and unexpected situations.

Along the way, we'll remind you that no two pregnancies are alike, and that's okay. Your journey is unique, and so is your baby.

A Few Words of Encouragement

You don't need to have all the answers right now. Every step you take, every choice you make, and every moment you spend preparing for your baby is a step toward being the incredible parent you're destined to be.

So, take a deep breath. Let's explore the beautiful, unpredictable, and extraordinary world of pregnancy together. This is your story, and it's just beginning.

Chapter 1: Understanding Pregnancy

What Happens When You're Pregnant

Pregnancy is an incredible process where a tiny fertilized egg grows into a fully developed baby over approximately 40 weeks. This journey is divided into three stages called trimesters, each marked by specific milestones and changes in your body and your baby's development.

From the moment of conception, your body begins to adapt to support the new life growing inside you. Hormones surge, organs adjust, and your body transforms in extraordinary ways. Understanding these changes can help you feel more in tune with your body and what's happening inside it.

Key Pregnancy Stages: Trimester by Trimester

First Trimester (Weeks 1–12): The Foundation

This is the stage where it all begins. In the first trimester:

- **Your baby:** The fertilized egg implants into the uterus and begins to grow rapidly. By the end of this stage, your baby is about the size of a plum, with all major organs formed.

- **Your body:** You may experience nausea, fatigue, and heightened emotions as your body adjusts to new hormones. It's also a time for essential screenings and early prenatal care.

Second Trimester (Weeks 13–26): Growth and Energy

Often called the "golden period" of pregnancy, the second trimester is when many women feel their best:

- **Your baby**: By this stage, your baby is growing steadily, developing key features like fingerprints, and beginning to move, which you might start to feel around week 18–20.

- **Your body**: You may notice a baby bump forming, and symptoms like morning sickness often subside.

Third Trimester (Weeks 27–40): Preparing for Birth

The final stretch is all about growth and preparation:

- **Your baby**: Rapid growth continues, and your baby begins to develop fat layers for warmth. By week 37, they're considered full-term and ready for the outside world.

- **Your body**: You may experience backaches, swelling, and the anticipation of labor as your due date approaches.

Understanding Your Baby's Development

From a single cell to a baby capable of surviving in the outside world, your baby undergoes remarkable changes:

- **Heartbeat**: By week 6, the tiny heart starts beating.

- **Senses**: Eyes, ears, and taste buds begin to develop by the second trimester.

- **Brain Growth**: Your baby's brain grows rapidly in the third trimester, setting the stage for learning and memory after birth.

Your Emotional Journey

Pregnancy isn't just a physical experience—it's an emotional one, too. You may feel everything from joy and excitement to worry and self-doubt. These feelings are completely normal. A strong support system and open communication with your healthcare provider can make all the difference.

Chapter 2 : Preparing for Pregnancy

Preconception Health Tips

Preparing for pregnancy starts long before you see a positive test result. Taking steps to optimize your health now can make a significant difference in your pregnancy journey and your baby's development.

- **Schedule a Preconception Checkup**: Visit your healthcare provider to discuss your plans. They may suggest vaccines, tests, or managing existing health conditions.

- **Start Taking Prenatal Vitamins**: Folic acid is crucial to prevent neural tube defects. Begin taking a prenatal vitamin with at least 400 mcg of folic acid three months before trying to conceive.

- **Quit Harmful Habits**: If you smoke, drink alcohol, or use drugs, now is the time to stop. These can negatively impact fertility and your baby's health.

- **Review Medications**: Consult your doctor about any prescriptions or over-the-counter medications you're taking to ensure they're safe for pregnancy.

Nutrition and Fitness Before Pregnancy

A balanced diet and regular exercise can boost your fertility and prepare your body for the physical demands of pregnancy.

- **Healthy Eating**:

  - Focus on whole grains, lean proteins, healthy fats, and plenty of fruits and vegetables.

  - Avoid high-mercury fish and limit caffeine.

- **Hydration**: Drink plenty of water daily to maintain optimal health.

- **Exercise**: Engage in moderate physical activity like walking, swimming, or yoga. Regular exercise can improve circulation, reduce stress, and prepare your body for labor.

Managing Preexisting Conditions

If you have chronic conditions such as diabetes, hypertension, or thyroid disorders, work closely with your doctor to stabilize them before conception. Proper management can reduce risks for both you and your baby.

- **Diabetes**: Keep blood sugar levels under control.

- **Hypertension**: Monitor blood pressure and discuss safe medications.

- **Mental Health**: Address anxiety or depression with a healthcare provider. Pregnancy can amplify these conditions, so early intervention is essential.

Understanding Your Fertility

Knowing how your menstrual cycle works can increase your chances of conceiving:

- **Track Ovulation**: Ovulation typically occurs about 14 days before your next period. Apps, ovulation predictor kits, or basal body temperature monitoring can help pinpoint your fertile window.

- **Maintain a Healthy Weight**: Being underweight or overweight can affect ovulation and fertility.

Lifestyle Adjustments for Both Partners

Preparing for pregnancy isn't just about the mother—it's a team effort.

- **For You**: Prioritize self-care and reduce stress.

- **For Your Partner**: Encourage healthy habits like a balanced diet, regular exercise, and avoiding tobacco and excessive alcohol, as these can impact sperm quality.

Emotional and Financial Preparation

Pregnancy brings emotional and financial changes. Taking steps to prepare now can ease the transition:

- **Emotional Readiness**: Discuss your expectations and fears with your partner or support system. Consider journaling or speaking with a counselor if needed.

- **Financial Planning**: Review your budget and research maternity leave policies, childcare costs, and insurance coverage for prenatal and delivery care.

Chapter 3: The First Trimester

What to Expect: Physical and Emotional Changes

The first trimester (weeks 1–12) is a period of rapid change, both for you and your growing baby. While it's an exciting time, it can also be challenging as your body adapts to pregnancy.

- **Physical Changes:**
    - **Fatigue:** Hormonal shifts and increased energy demands can leave you feeling tired. Rest whenever possible.
    - **Morning Sickness:** Nausea, often triggered by certain smells or foods, is common. Despite the name, it can occur any time of day.
    - **Breast Tenderness:** Hormonal changes may make your breasts feel sore or swollen.
    - **Frequent Urination:** Your growing uterus and increased blood flow may lead to more bathroom trips.

- **Emotional Changes:**
    - Hormonal fluctuations might make you feel moody or emotional.
    - Excitement and anxiety about the baby's health are normal. Share your feelings with loved ones or a healthcare provider if they become overwhelming.

Essential Tests and Appointments

Your first prenatal visit is crucial for establishing care and setting the foundation for a healthy pregnancy. During this visit, you can expect:

- **Health History Review**: Your doctor will ask about your medical history, lifestyle, and any previous pregnancies.

- **Ultrasound**: Often performed around 6–8 weeks to confirm the pregnancy and check your baby's heartbeat.

- **Routine Blood Tests**: To check your blood type, Rh factor, and screen for anemia, infections, and immunity to certain diseases like rubella.

- **Genetic Testing Options**: Tests like the NIPT (non-invasive prenatal testing) can screen for chromosomal conditions like Down syndrome.

Coping with Morning Sickness

Morning sickness affects up to 70% of pregnant women. Here are some tips to ease symptoms:

- **Eat Small, Frequent Meals**: Keeping your stomach slightly full can help.

- **Stay Hydrated**: Sip water, ginger tea, or electrolyte drinks.

- **Avoid Triggers**: Identify and steer clear of foods or smells that worsen your nausea.

- **Consult Your Doctor**: If nausea becomes severe (hyperemesis gravidarum), your doctor can recommend safe treatments.

Your Baby's Development in the First Trimester

Your baby grows from a tiny ball of cells to a recognizable fetus by the end of this trimester:

- **Weeks 1–4**: The fertilized egg implants in the uterus. The neural tube, which becomes the brain and spinal cord, begins forming.

- **Weeks 5–8**: Major organs like the heart, liver, and kidneys start to develop. Your baby's heartbeat can often be detected via ultrasound.

- **Weeks 9–12**: The face becomes more defined, tiny limbs form, and the baby begins to move (though you likely won't feel it yet).

Tips for Self-Care

- **Rest**: Listen to your body and take naps or relax when needed.

- **Nutrition**: Focus on eating nutrient-rich foods and avoiding raw fish, unpasteurized dairy, and high-mercury fish.

- **Stay Active**: Light exercises like walking or prenatal yoga can improve circulation and boost energy.

- **Communicate**: Share your experiences and concerns with your partner or support system.

When to Call Your Doctor

Contact your healthcare provider if you experience:

- Heavy bleeding or severe cramping.

- Persistent nausea and vomiting that prevents you from eating or drinking.

- High fever or unusual pain.

Chapter 4: The Second Trimester

What to Expect: Physical and Emotional Changes

The second trimester (weeks 13–26) is often considered the most enjoyable phase of pregnancy. Many early symptoms, like nausea and fatigue, subside, and you may feel more energetic and excited.

- **Physical Changes**:

    - **Baby Bump**: Your belly becomes more noticeable as your baby grows.

    - **Increased Appetite**: With morning sickness fading, you might feel hungrier.

    - **Skin Changes**: Hormonal shifts may cause a "pregnancy glow" or lead to stretch marks and darkened patches of skin.

    - **Movements**: You may feel your baby's first flutters, known as "quickening," around 18–22 weeks.

- **Emotional Changes**:

    - You might feel a deeper connection with your baby as movements become more noticeable.

    - Concerns about labor, delivery, or parenting may arise—perfectly normal as you prepare for this life-changing event.

Growth and Development of Your Baby

During the second trimester, your baby undergoes remarkable changes:

- **Weeks 13–16**: The skeleton hardens, and facial features become more defined.

- **Weeks 17–20**: Your baby can hear sounds and even respond to your voice.

- **Weeks 21–26**: The lungs and digestive system continue to mature, and your baby begins to develop a sleep-wake cycle.

By the end of this trimester, your baby is around 14 inches long and weighs about 1.5 pounds.

Medical Appointments and Tests

The second trimester includes key medical checkups and screenings:

- **Ultrasound Anatomy Scan** (around 20 weeks): This detailed scan checks your baby's growth, development, and gender (if you choose to find out).

- **Gestational Diabetes Test** (around 24–28 weeks): A glucose tolerance test to ensure your body processes sugar effectively.

- **Blood Pressure Monitoring**: Regular checks for signs of preeclampsia.

Dealing with Body Changes

Your body is adapting rapidly. Here's how to manage common discomforts:

- **Back Pain**: Use proper posture and consider a maternity support belt.

- **Heartburn**: Eat smaller meals and avoid spicy or greasy foods.

- **Leg Cramps**: Stay hydrated and stretch before bed.

- **Swelling**: Elevate your feet when resting and wear comfortable shoes.

Planning Your Maternity Leave

If you're employed, now is the time to discuss maternity leave with your employer. Consider:

- **Leave Policies**: Understand your company's policies and your country's laws regarding maternity leave.

- **Finances**: Plan your budget for the time you'll be off work.

- **Work Handover**: Begin organizing tasks and training a colleague if needed.

Connecting with Your Baby

Bonding with your baby during this trimester can be deeply rewarding:

- Talk or sing to your baby—they can hear your voice.

- Attend prenatal classes to prepare for childbirth and parenting.

- Start thinking about baby names, nursery decor, and the essentials you'll need after birth.

Chapter 5: The Third Trimester

What to Expect: Physical and Emotional Changes

The third trimester (weeks 27–40) is the final stage of your pregnancy journey. While excitement builds as you prepare to meet your baby, this period can also bring physical discomfort and emotional ups and downs.

- **Physical Changes:**

  - **Rapid Baby Growth:** Your baby is gaining weight quickly, which may increase pressure on your back, pelvis, and bladder.

  - **Braxton Hicks Contractions:** These "practice contractions" can cause mild, irregular tightening in your abdomen.

  - **Swelling:** It's common in the feet, ankles, and hands due to increased fluid retention.

  - **Shortness of Breath:** As your uterus expands, it may press on your diaphragm.

- **Emotional Changes:**

  - You may feel impatient or anxious about labor and delivery.

  - A mix of excitement and apprehension about becoming a parent is natural.

Preparing for Labor and Delivery

As your due date approaches, focus on getting ready for the big day:

- **Learn the Signs of Labor**:

    - Regular contractions that increase in intensity and frequency.

    - Loss of the mucus plug or water breaking.

    - A persistent lower backache or pelvic pressure.

- **Choose Your Birth Plan**:

    - Decide where you want to give birth (hospital, birthing center, or home).

    - Discuss pain management options, like epidurals or natural techniques, with your healthcare provider.

- **Take a Prenatal Class**: Many hospitals offer classes on childbirth, breastfeeding, and newborn care.

Common Discomforts and Remedies

The third trimester can be physically challenging. Here's how to ease discomfort:

- **Back Pain**: Sleep with a pillow between your knees and try prenatal massages.

- **Insomnia**: Practice relaxation techniques and create a bedtime routine.

- **Heartburn**: Avoid large meals before bed and sleep propped up with pillows.

- **Frequent Urination**: Plan bathroom breaks and stay hydrated during the day rather than late at night.

Packing Your Hospital Bag

Packing early ensures you're ready when labor begins. Essentials include:

- **For You**: Comfortable clothes, toiletries, and any personal items like a phone charger or birth plan.

- **For Baby**: A going-home outfit, diapers, and a blanket.

- **For Your Partner**: Snacks, a change of clothes, and a list of important contacts.

Your Baby's Development

By the third trimester, your baby is almost fully formed and focused on preparing for life outside the womb:

- **Weeks 27–30**: The baby's eyes open, and they begin responding to light and sound.

- **Weeks 31–34**: Fat stores build, and the baby practices breathing by inhaling amniotic fluid.

- **Weeks 35–40**: The baby gains the most weight, typically reaching 6–9 pounds. They settle into a head-down position in preparation for birth.

Caring for Your Emotional Well-Being

The anticipation of childbirth can bring a mix of emotions. To stay balanced:

- **Stay Informed**: Learn about labor stages and pain relief options.

- **Ask for Support**: Share your thoughts and feelings with your partner or a trusted friend.

- **Practice Relaxation**: Breathing exercises, meditation, or gentle yoga can help ease anxiety.

Chapter 6: Nutrition During Pregnancy

The Importance of a Balanced Diet

Eating well during pregnancy is one of the best things you can do for yourself and your growing baby. A nutrient-rich diet supports your baby's development while keeping your energy levels steady and your body strong.

- **Focus on Variety**: Include a mix of fruits, vegetables, whole grains, lean proteins, and healthy fats.

- **Quality Over Quantity**: While you'll need more calories, it's about nourishing your body with quality foods rather than eating for two.

Essential Nutrients for Pregnancy

Certain nutrients play a critical role in supporting a healthy pregnancy:

- **Folic Acid**: Helps prevent neural tube defects. Found in leafy greens, fortified cereals, and prenatal vitamins.

- **Iron**: Supports increased blood volume and prevents anemia. Found in lean meats, spinach, and legumes. Pair with vitamin C for better absorption.

- **Calcium**: Essential for your baby's bone and teeth development. Found in dairy products, almonds, and fortified plant-based milk.

- **DHA (Omega-3 Fatty Acids)**: Aids in your baby's brain and eye development. Found in fatty fish like salmon and walnuts.

- **Protein**: Crucial for cell growth and repair. Found in eggs, chicken, tofu, and beans.

Foods to Avoid

To protect your baby from potential harm, steer clear of:

- **Raw or Undercooked Foods**: Sushi, rare meats, and soft-boiled eggs may harbor bacteria or parasites.

- **High-Mercury Fish**: Limit swordfish, king mackerel, and tilefish.

- **Unpasteurized Products**: Avoid unpasteurized milk, cheeses, and juices.

- **Excessive Caffeine**: Limit to 200 mg per day (about one 12-ounce cup of coffee).

- **Alcohol**: No amount is considered safe during pregnancy.

Managing Pregnancy Cravings and Aversions

It's normal to crave certain foods or feel repulsed by others during pregnancy. Here's how to handle them:

- **Cravings**: If cravings are for healthy foods, enjoy them in moderation. For less healthy options, find healthier alternatives or indulge occasionally without guilt.

- **Aversions**: Focus on foods you can tolerate while ensuring you meet your nutritional needs.

Staying Hydrated

Hydration is just as important as eating well:

- **Daily Water Intake**: Aim for at least 8–10 glasses of water a day.

- **Healthy Hydration Alternatives**: Try herbal teas, smoothies, or infused water with fruits and herbs.

Supplements: Filling the Gaps

While a healthy diet covers most of your nutritional needs, prenatal vitamins provide an extra boost:

- **Prenatal Multivitamins**: Ensure you're getting enough folic acid, iron, calcium, and DHA.

- **Discuss with Your Doctor**: Avoid megadoses or additional supplements unless prescribed.

Sample Meal Plan for a Day

Here's an example of a balanced day of eating:

✓ **Breakfast**: Whole-grain toast with avocado, a boiled egg, and a glass of orange juice.

✓ **Snack**: Greek yogurt with fresh berries and a handful of nuts.

✓ **Lunch**: Grilled chicken salad with mixed greens, quinoa, and a vinaigrette dressing.

✓ **Snack**: A banana with a tablespoon of almond butter.

✓ **Dinner**: Baked salmon, roasted sweet potatoes, and steamed broccoli.

✓ **Dessert**: A small bowl of dark chocolate and strawberries.

Special Considerations

- **Gestational Diabetes**: If diagnosed, work with a dietitian to manage blood sugar levels through diet.

- **Vegetarian or Vegan Diets**: Ensure adequate protein, iron, and B12 intake. Speak to your doctor about supplements if needed.

Chapter 7: Exercise and Staying Active During Pregnancy

The Benefits of Exercise During Pregnancy

Staying active during pregnancy is beneficial for both you and your baby. Regular physical activity can:

- Improve mood and energy levels.

- Reduce common discomforts like back pain and swelling.

- Help maintain a healthy weight gain.

- Prepare your body for labor and delivery by improving strength and endurance.

- Lower the risk of gestational diabetes and preeclampsia.

Safe Exercises for Each Trimester

While exercise is generally safe during pregnancy, it's essential to adapt your routine to your changing body.

- **First Trimester:**

  - Focus on low-impact exercises like walking, swimming, or prenatal yoga.

  - Avoid activities with a high risk of falling or abdominal trauma, like skiing or contact sports.

- **Second Trimester:**

  - As your baby bump grows, prioritize balance and stability. Try stationary cycling, water aerobics, or light strength training.

  - Avoid lying flat on your back for extended periods, as it can reduce blood flow to your baby.

- **Third Trimester:**

  - Gentle stretching and relaxation exercises like prenatal yoga or Pilates can ease tension and prepare your body for labor.

  - Short walks or swimming can help maintain mobility and circulation.

Listening to Your Body

It's crucial to pay attention to how you feel during and after exercise. Stop immediately and contact your doctor if you experience:

- Vaginal bleeding or fluid leakage.

- Dizziness or feeling faint.

- Shortness of breath before starting activity.

- Severe abdominal or pelvic pain.

- Uterine contractions or reduced baby movements.

Tips for Staying Active Safely

1. **Get Medical Clearance**: Always check with your healthcare provider before starting or continuing an exercise program.

2. **Warm-Up and Cool Down**: Prepare your body for activity and prevent soreness by including 5–10 minutes of light stretching.

3. **Stay Hydrated**: Drink plenty of water before, during, and after exercise to avoid dehydration.

4. **Wear Supportive Gear**: Choose comfortable, breathable clothing and a supportive sports bra. Consider wearing maternity support belts as your belly grows.

5. **Avoid Overheating**: Exercise in a cool, well-ventilated area and avoid hot yoga or strenuous workouts in high temperatures.

Pelvic Floor Exercises: A Must-Do

Strengthening your pelvic floor muscles is vital for pregnancy and postpartum recovery.

- **Kegel Exercises**: Contract and hold the pelvic muscles for a few seconds, then release. Repeat 10–15 times daily to reduce the risk of incontinence and support delivery.

Staying Motivated

- Join a prenatal fitness class to connect with other pregnant women.

- Set small, achievable goals to maintain consistency.

- Focus on activities you enjoy to make exercising more fun.

When to Modify or Stop Exercise

Your body will signal when it's time to slow down. Modifications may be necessary if you experience:

- Increased fatigue or persistent soreness after workouts.

- Balance issues or discomfort during certain movements.

Special Considerations

- **High-Risk Pregnancies**: If you have conditions like placenta previa, preeclampsia, or preterm labor risk, consult your doctor before exercising.

- **Previously Inactive Moms**: Start slow with light activities like walking or stretching, gradually increasing intensity.

Chapter 8: Common Pregnancy Challenges and How to Manage Them

Pregnancy is an incredible journey, but it can also come with physical and emotional challenges. Knowing how to navigate these difficulties can help you stay comfortable and confident throughout the process.

- **Physical Challenges**

1. **Morning Sickness**

   - **Symptoms**: Nausea and vomiting, especially during the first trimester.

   - **Solutions**:

     - Eat small, frequent meals.

     - Keep crackers or dry snacks by your bedside.

     - Sip ginger tea or try ginger candies.

     - Consult your doctor if symptoms are severe.

2. **Fatigue**

- **Symptoms**: Feeling excessively tired, particularly in the first and third trimesters.

- **Solutions**:

  - Rest when you need to.

  - Incorporate iron-rich foods into your diet to prevent anemia.

  - Stay hydrated and engage in light exercise for an energy boost.

3. **Heartburn and Indigestion**

- **Symptoms**: Burning sensation in the chest or discomfort after eating.

- **Solutions**:

    - Avoid spicy, greasy, or acidic foods.

    - Eat slowly and chew thoroughly.

    - Stay upright for at least an hour after meals.

    - Ask your doctor about antacids if needed.

4. **Back Pain**

- **Symptoms**: Aches or sharp pain in the lower back.

- **Solutions**:

    - Use a maternity support belt.

    - Practice good posture and avoid standing for long periods.

    - Try prenatal yoga or stretches designed for back pain relief.

5. **Swelling (Edema)**

- **Symptoms**: Swollen feet, ankles, or hands.

- **Solutions**:

    - Elevate your feet when sitting.

    - Wear compression stockings.

    - Drink plenty of water to flush excess fluids.

    - Avoid standing for prolonged periods.

6. **Leg Cramps**

- **Symptoms**: Sudden, sharp pains in the legs, often at night.

- **Solutions**:

  - Stretch your calves before bed.

  - Stay hydrated and maintain a balanced intake of calcium and magnesium.

  - Massage the area and apply heat if cramps occur.

Emotional Challenges

1. **Mood Swings**

- **Causes**: Hormonal changes, stress, and physical discomfort.

- **Solutions**:

  - Practice relaxation techniques like meditation or deep breathing.

  - Talk to a trusted friend, partner, or therapist.

  - Ensure you're getting enough rest and eating well.

2. **Anxiety About Labor and Delivery**

- **Causes**: Fear of pain, complications, or the unknown.

- **Solutions**:

  - Attend childbirth education classes.

  - Learn relaxation techniques for labor, like breathing exercises.

  - Speak openly with your healthcare provider about your concerns.

3. **Body Image Concerns**

- **Causes**: Changes in weight and body shape.

- **Solutions**:

    - Focus on the amazing work your body is doing to grow your baby.

    - Stay active and eat nutritious foods to feel your best.

    - Connect with other moms to share experiences and encouragement.

Serious Complications: Know the Warning Signs

While most pregnancy symptoms are normal, some can indicate serious issues. Contact your doctor if you experience:

- Heavy bleeding or severe abdominal pain.

- Sudden, severe swelling, especially in the face or hands.

- Persistent headaches or vision changes.

- Decreased baby movements after 28 weeks.

- High fever or flu-like symptoms.

Building a Support System

Don't hesitate to ask for help when you need it:

- **Partner Support**: Involve your partner in appointments, prenatal classes, and preparations.

- **Family and Friends**: Let them assist with household tasks, meals, or errands.

- **Professional Support**: Consider joining a pregnancy support group or talking to a counselor.

Chapter 9: Building a Strong Support System

Having a reliable support system during pregnancy can make your journey smoother, less stressful, and more enjoyable. A strong network provides emotional reassurance, practical help, and invaluable advice as you prepare for parenthood.

Why a Support System Matters

Pregnancy comes with its ups and downs, and having supportive people around you can:

- Reduce stress and anxiety.

- Provide help with daily tasks.

- Offer a sense of community and understanding.

- Enhance your overall well-being.

Key Members of Your Support System

1. **Partner or Spouse**

    - Your partner can be your greatest source of support during pregnancy.

    - Ways they can help:

        - Attend prenatal appointments with you.

        - Participate in childbirth classes.

        - Share household responsibilities to ease your workload.

2. **Family and Friends**

   - Lean on family and friends for emotional support, advice, and practical help.

   - Examples:

     - A trusted friend to accompany you to appointments.

     - Family members to help with cooking, cleaning, or running errands.

3. **Healthcare Providers**

   - Your doctor, midwife, or obstetrician will guide you through the medical aspects of pregnancy.

   - Build a relationship where you feel comfortable asking questions or voicing concerns.

4. **Other Moms and Moms-to-Be**

   - Connecting with women who are pregnant or have recently given birth can be comforting.

   - Join local or online pregnancy support groups to share experiences and advice.

5. **Prenatal Instructors**

   - Prenatal yoga or childbirth education instructors can provide physical and emotional guidance as you prepare for delivery.

Building and Strengthening Your Support Network

1. **Communicate Your Needs**

   - Be open about what you need, whether it's a listening ear, help with chores, or advice.

   - Let people know how they can best support you.

2. **Attend Prenatal Classes**

   - Classes on childbirth, breastfeeding, or newborn care are great ways to involve your partner and meet other expecting parents.

3. **Join Online Communities**

   - Pregnancy forums and social media groups offer round-the-clock support and a wealth of shared knowledge.

4. **Set Boundaries**

   - Not all advice or help will be beneficial. Politely decline unsolicited opinions or assistance that doesn't feel right for you.

5. **Celebrate Your Journey Together**

   - Share milestones like baby's first kicks, ultrasound photos, or gender reveals with your support network to strengthen connections.

Professional Support Options

Sometimes you may need support beyond your immediate circle:

- **Therapists or Counselors**: If you're experiencing anxiety or depression, seek help from a mental health professional.

- **Lactation Consultants**: They can help you prepare for breastfeeding and address concerns after birth.

- **Doulas**: Hiring a doula provides continuous emotional and physical support during labor and delivery.

Self-Support: Being Your Own Advocate

While a support system is vital, it's equally important to advocate for yourself:

- Stay informed about your pregnancy and options for labor and delivery.

- Practice self-care by prioritizing rest, nutrition, and relaxation.

- Trust your instincts—if something doesn't feel right, speak up.

Chapter 10: Preparing for the Baby's Arrival

As your due date approaches, preparing for your baby's arrival becomes more exciting—and sometimes overwhelming. Breaking tasks into manageable steps can help you feel ready to welcome your little one.

Setting Up the Nursery

1. **Essential Furniture and Items:**

    - **Crib or Bassinet**: Ensure it meets current safety standards.

    - **Changing Table or Station**: A designated spot for diaper changes.

    - **Rocking Chair or Glider**: For feeding and soothing your baby.

    - **Storage**: Shelves or drawers for clothes, diapers, and baby supplies.

2. **Safety Measures:**

    - Use a firm mattress with a fitted sheet in the crib.

    - Avoid pillows, blankets, or stuffed toys in the crib to reduce the risk of suffocation.

    - Anchor heavy furniture to the wall to prevent tipping.

3. **Decorating the Space:**

    - Choose calming colors and themes.

    - Opt for washable and non-toxic materials.

Stocking Up on Baby Essentials

1. **Clothing**:

    - Onesies, sleepers, and socks (newborn and 0–3 months sizes).

    - Hats and mittens to keep your baby warm and scratch-free.

2. **Diapering Supplies**:

    - Diapers (newborn size) and wipes.

    - Diaper rash cream.

    - A diaper pail or disposal system.

3. **Feeding Supplies**:

    - If breastfeeding: Nursing bras, breast pump, milk storage bags, and nipple cream.

    - If formula feeding: Bottles, nipples, and formula.

4. **Bathing and Hygiene**:

    - Baby bathtub, gentle soap, and shampoo.

    - Soft towels and washcloths.

    - Baby nail clippers and a brush or comb.

5. **Travel and On-the-Go Items**:

    - A car seat (installed and checked for safety).

    - A sturdy stroller or baby carrier.

    - A well-organized diaper bag.

Packing Your Hospital Bag

Start packing around week 34 to ensure you're ready. Include:

- **For You**: Comfortable clothes, slippers, toiletries, and personal items (phone charger, birth plan).

- **For Baby**: A going-home outfit, a blanket, and a hat.

- **For Your Partner**: Snacks, a change of clothes, and entertainment like books or headphones.

Creating a Birth Plan

Your birth plan outlines your preferences for labor and delivery. Key elements to consider:

1. **Pain Management**: Decide if you want an epidural, natural techniques, or other options.

2. **Labor Preferences**: Positions for labor, mobility, and who you want in the delivery room.

3. **Post-Birth Care**: Immediate skin-to-skin contact, delayed cord clamping, or specific feeding preferences.

Discuss your birth plan with your healthcare provider to ensure it aligns with hospital policies.

Babyproofing Your Home

While your baby won't be mobile for a few months, it's helpful to start early:

- Install outlet covers and cabinet locks.

- Secure cords, blinds, and small objects that pose choking hazards.

- Ensure smoke and carbon monoxide detectors are functional.

Preparing Siblings and Pets

1. **For Siblings**:

   - Involve them in the preparations, such as setting up the nursery.

   - Read books or watch videos about becoming an older sibling.

   - Spend one-on-one time with them to reassure them of their importance.

2. **For Pets**:

   - Introduce them to baby sounds and scents in advance.

   - Set boundaries for areas like the nursery.

   - Gradually adjust their routine to match the baby's schedule.

Emotional Preparation for Parenthood

1. **Build Confidence**: Educate yourself through parenting classes or books.

2. **Discuss Expectations**: Talk openly with your partner about parenting roles and responsibilities.

3. **Anticipate Challenges**: Understand that the early days may be exhausting but are also rewarding.

Final Checklist Before the Baby Arrives

- Confirm your hospital route and practice the drive.

- Install the car seat correctly.

- Schedule a prenatal check-up for a final assessment.

- Arrange for help during the postpartum period, whether from family, friends, or a postpartum doula.

By preparing thoroughly, you can ease your transition into parenthood and focus on the joy of welcoming your baby.

Chapter 11: Labor and Delivery

The arrival of your baby is an exciting and transformative moment. Understanding what to expect during labor and delivery can ease your mind and help you feel more prepared for this life-changing experience.

Understanding the Stages of Labor

Labor is divided into three main stages:

1. **First Stage: Early Labor and Active Labor**

   - **Early Labor:**

     - Cervix begins to dilate (up to 4 cm).

     - Contractions are mild and irregular, lasting 30–45 seconds and spaced 20–30 minutes apart.

     - What to Do: Stay home, rest, eat light snacks, and keep hydrated. Use relaxation techniques or take a warm bath.

   - **Active Labor:**

     - Cervix dilates from 4 to 10 cm.

     - Contractions become stronger, longer (45–60 seconds), and closer together (3–5 minutes apart).

     - What to Do: Go to the hospital or birthing center. Focus on breathing exercises and pain management strategies.

2. **Second Stage: Pushing and Delivery**

   - **Duration**: A few minutes to several hours.

   - **What Happens**:

     - Your cervix is fully dilated.

     - You'll feel a strong urge to push as your baby moves through the birth canal.

     - Your baby is born!

   - **Tips**:

     - Follow your doctor or midwife's instructions to push effectively.

     - Use upright positions like squatting or leaning to leverage gravity.

3. **Third Stage: Delivery of the Placenta**

   - **Duration**: Typically 5–30 minutes after the baby is born.

   - **What Happens**: The placenta detaches from the uterine wall and is delivered.

   - **Tips**: Relax and enjoy your first moments with your baby while your doctor monitors you for bleeding.

Signs That Labor Is Starting

- Regular contractions that get closer together and increase in intensity.

- Lower back pain or cramping that doesn't go away.

- A bloody or mucus-like discharge (the "bloody show").

- Water breaking (a gush or trickle of amniotic fluid).

If you experience any of these signs, contact your healthcare provider.

Pain Management During Labor

You have several options for managing pain during labor:

1. **Natural Techniques**:

    - Breathing exercises, visualization, and relaxation techniques.

    - Using a birthing ball, warm showers, or massages.

    - Partner support and encouragement.

2. **Medical Options**:

    - **Epidural**: Provides significant pain relief by numbing the lower half of your body.

    - **IV Pain Medication**: Offers temporary relief but doesn't eliminate all sensation.

Discuss these options with your doctor in advance to choose what feels right for you.

Delivery Methods

1. **Vaginal Delivery**:

    - The most common method.

    - Can be unmedicated or include pain relief like an epidural.

2. **Cesarean Section (C-Section)**:

    - A surgical procedure where the baby is delivered through an incision in the abdomen.

    - May be planned or performed as an emergency procedure if complications arise.

3. **Assisted Delivery:**

   - Tools like forceps or a vacuum may be used to help guide the baby out during vaginal delivery if needed.

Role of Your Support Team

- **Partner**: Provide emotional support, massage, or help with breathing exercises.

- **Doula**: Offer continuous physical and emotional support during labor.

- **Medical Team**: Ensure the safety and health of you and your baby throughout the process.

Post-Delivery Care

1. **Immediate Skin-to-Skin Contact:**

   - Promotes bonding and stabilizes your baby's temperature and heart rate.

2. **Breastfeeding Initiation:**

   - Encourage your baby to latch within the first hour if possible.

3. **Monitoring:**

   - Your doctor will check for excessive bleeding and help you recover from delivery.

Emotional Aspects of Labor and Delivery

- It's normal to feel a mix of emotions—excitement, fear, and relief.

- Trust your body and your support team. Remember, every labor is unique, and your experience will be, too.

Chapter 12: Postpartum Recovery and Care

The postpartum period, often referred to as the "fourth trimester," is a time of significant physical, emotional, and lifestyle adjustment. Proper care for yourself during this time is essential as you recover from childbirth and adapt to your new role as a parent.

- **Physical Recovery After Childbirth**

1. **Vaginal Birth Recovery**

    - **Healing**: It's normal to experience vaginal soreness, swelling, or minor tears.

    - **Tips for Comfort:**

        - Use cold packs or sitz baths to reduce swelling.

        - Take pain relievers as recommended by your doctor.

        - Practice gentle Kegel exercises to strengthen pelvic muscles.

2. **C-Section Recovery**

    - **Healing**: Recovery from a cesarean section typically takes longer than vaginal birth.

    - **Tips for Comfort:**

        - Keep the incision clean and dry.

        - Avoid heavy lifting and strenuous activities for at least 6–8 weeks.

        - Take prescribed pain medications and follow up with your doctor for wound checks.

3. **Managing Bleeding**

   - Expect postpartum bleeding (lochia) for several weeks, which starts heavy and gradually decreases.

   - Use sanitary pads instead of tampons to avoid infection.

4. **Dealing with Breast Changes**

   - You may experience engorgement, leaking, or sore nipples, especially when breastfeeding.

   - **Tips**:

     - Use warm compresses to ease engorgement.

     - Apply nipple cream to soothe soreness.

     - Wear a supportive bra to reduce discomfort.

Emotional Recovery

1. **Postpartum Emotions**

   - Hormonal changes can lead to mood swings, irritability, or "baby blues," which typically resolve within two weeks.

   - Seek support from your partner, family, or a therapist if needed.

2. **Postpartum Depression (PPD)**

   - **Signs**: Persistent sadness, withdrawal, anxiety, or difficulty bonding with your baby.

   - **What to Do**: Talk to your healthcare provider for treatment options, including therapy or medication.

3. **Adjusting to Parenthood**

   - It's natural to feel overwhelmed. Focus on small victories and allow yourself time to learn.

Establishing a Routine

1. **Sleep**

   - Sleep deprivation is common. Rest when the baby sleeps and share nighttime duties with your partner.

2. **Nutrition**

   - Focus on nutrient-rich foods to aid recovery. Include lean protein, whole grains, fruits, vegetables, and plenty of fluids.

3. **Physical Activity**

   - Begin light activities, like walking, as you feel able. Avoid strenuous exercises until cleared by your doctor.

Breastfeeding and Bottle-Feeding

1. **Breastfeeding**

   - Benefits: Provides optimal nutrition and strengthens the bond between mother and baby.
   - Seek help from a lactation consultant if you encounter challenges like latching issues or low milk supply.

2. **Bottle-Feeding**

   - Use formula or pumped breast milk. Sterilize bottles and nipples to ensure cleanliness.

Caring for Your Mental Health

- Take time for yourself, even if it's just a few quiet minutes each day.

- Don't hesitate to ask for help with household tasks or baby care.

- Join a new moms' support group to share experiences and build connections

Postpartum Doctor Visits

1. **Six-Week Check-Up**

   - Your healthcare provider will check your recovery, address concerns, and discuss contraception or family planning.

2. **Follow-Up for C-Section**

   - Additional appointments may be required to monitor incision healing.

Balancing Parenthood and Relationships

- Communication is key with your partner. Share responsibilities and express your feelings openly.

- Schedule moments to reconnect as a couple, even amidst the chaos of caring for a newborn.

Remember to Celebrate Your Journey

Postpartum recovery is a gradual process. Be kind to yourself, and remember that every parent's experience is unique. Celebrate the small milestones, and cherish the precious moments with your baby.

Chapter 13: Baby's First Year: What to Expect

Your baby's first year is a time of rapid growth and change. Understanding what to expect in terms of development, milestones, and caregiving can help you navigate this exciting journey with confidence.

- **Key Developmental Milestones**

- **Physical Development**

  - **0–3 Months:**

    - Gains head control and begins to follow objects with their eyes.

    - Reflexes like grasping and rooting are prominent.

  - **4–6 Months:**

    - Rolls over, begins to sit with support, and may start teething.

    - Reaches for and grasps objects.

  - **7–9 Months:**

    - Sits without support, crawls, and may pull to stand.

    - Transfers objects between hands.

  - **10–12 Months:**

    - Takes first steps or cruises along furniture.

    - Begins to use the pincer grasp (thumb and forefinger).

2. **Cognitive Development**

   - Shows curiosity about the environment.

   - Learns to recognize faces and objects.

   - Develops problem-solving skills, such as figuring out how to reach a toy.

3. **Social and Emotional Development**

   - Smiles in response to others (social smile).

   - Develops attachment to caregivers and may experience stranger anxiety.

   - Enjoys interactive games like peek-a-boo.

4. **Language Development**

   - **0–3 Months**: Responds to sounds and coos.

   - **4–6 Months**: Starts babbling and mimicking sounds.

   - **7–12 Months**: Says simple words like "mama" or "dada" and responds to their name.

Feeding Your Baby

1. **Breastfeeding or Formula Feeding**

   - **0–6 Months**: Breast milk or formula provides all the nutrition your baby needs.

   - Feed on demand, typically every 2–4 hours.

2. **Introducing Solids**

   - **Around 6 Months**: Begin with pureed fruits, vegetables, or iron-fortified cereals.

   - Gradually introduce new foods one at a time to monitor for allergies.

3. **Transitioning to Finger Foods**

   - **8–12 Months**: Offer small, soft pieces of food like banana slices or cooked vegetables.

   - Encourage self-feeding to develop coordination.

Sleep Patterns

1. **Newborns (0–3 Months)**

   - Sleep 14–17 hours a day in short intervals.

   - Establish a consistent sleep environment with a dark, quiet room and a safe crib.

2. **Infants (4–12 Months)**

   - Sleep consolidates into longer stretches at night, with 2–3 naps during the day.

   - Begin a bedtime routine, such as bathing, reading, or singing, to signal sleep time.

Health and Wellness

1. **Vaccinations**

    - Follow the recommended immunization schedule to protect your baby from illnesses.

2. **Doctor Visits**

    - Schedule regular well-baby check-ups to monitor growth and development.

3. **Illness Prevention**

    - Practice good hygiene and limit exposure to sick individuals.
    - Learn the signs of common illnesses, like fever or ear infections, and know when to call your doctor.

Encouraging Development Through Play

1. **Tummy Time**

    - Place your baby on their stomach daily to strengthen neck and upper body muscles.

2. **Interactive Toys and Games**

    - Offer toys that encourage grasping, shaking, or stacking.
    - Play peek-a-boo or sing nursery rhymes to engage your baby.

3. **Reading Together**

    - Introduce books early to stimulate language development and bonding.

Building a Strong Bond

1. **Skin-to-Skin Contact**

   - Continue skin-to-skin cuddling to provide comfort and security.

2. **Responding to Cues**

   - Pay attention to your baby's signals, such as hunger or sleepiness.

   - Comfort them promptly to build trust and attachment.

3. **Spending Quality Time**

   - Engage in eye contact, talk to your baby, and involve them in daily activities.

Challenges in the First Year

1. **Sleep Deprivation**

   - Share nighttime duties with your partner and prioritize rest when possible.

2. **Feeding Difficulties**

   - Seek support from a pediatrician or lactation consultant if breastfeeding or bottle-feeding issues arise.

3. **Parental Adjustment**

   - Remember, it's okay to ask for help and take breaks to recharge.

Cherishing the First Year

Your baby's first year will be filled with precious moments and milestones. Capture these memories through photos, journaling, or keepsakes. Celebrate the small victories and remember that every baby develops at their own pace.

Chapter 14: Common Pregnancy and Newborn Myths Debunked

Parenthood is often accompanied by a flood of advice—some helpful, some outdated, and some downright incorrect. This chapter addresses common myths about pregnancy and newborn care to help you make informed decisions.

Pregnancy Myths and Truths

1. **Myth: You Can't Exercise During Pregnancy**

   - **Truth**: Moderate exercise is generally safe and beneficial for most pregnancies. Activities like walking, swimming, or prenatal yoga can improve your mood, stamina, and overall health. Always consult your doctor before starting a new exercise routine.

2. **Myth: You're Eating for Two**

   - **Truth**: While your nutritional needs increase during pregnancy, you only need about 300 extra calories per day in the second and third trimesters. Focus on nutrient-dense foods rather than overeating.

3. **Myth: Morning Sickness Only Happens in the Morning**

   - **Truth**: Nausea can occur at any time of the day or night during pregnancy. Eating small, frequent meals and staying hydrated can help alleviate symptoms.

4. **Myth: The Shape of Your Belly Predicts Your Baby's Gender**

    - **Truth**: The shape of your belly is determined by your body type, muscle tone, and the baby's position, not their gender. Ultrasound or genetic testing is the only reliable way to determine gender.

5. **Myth: Spicy Foods or Pineapple Can Trigger Labor**

    - **Truth**: No scientific evidence supports the claim that specific foods induce labor. Labor typically begins when your baby is ready, and your body produces the necessary hormones.

Newborn Care Myths and Truths

1. **Myth: Picking Up Your Baby When They Cry Will Spoil Them**

   - **Truth**: Newborns cry to communicate needs like hunger, discomfort, or a desire for closeness. Responding promptly helps build trust and security. You can't spoil a baby by meeting their needs.

2. **Myth: Babies Should Sleep Through the Night by Three Months**

   - **Truth**: Sleep patterns vary widely. Many babies don't consistently sleep through the night until 6–12 months or later. Patience and a consistent bedtime routine can help improve sleep over time.

3. **Myth: You Must Sterilize Everything for Your Baby**

   - **Truth**: While it's essential to keep feeding equipment clean, daily sterilization isn't always necessary unless your baby is premature or has a weakened immune system. Regular washing with hot, soapy water is usually sufficient.

4. **Myth: Newborns Need Daily Baths**

   - **Truth**: Bathing your baby 2–3 times a week is sufficient. Overbathing can dry out their delicate skin. Focus on keeping the diaper area and folds of skin clean between baths.

5. **Myth: A Fever Always Means Illness**

   - **Truth**: A mild fever can be a normal response to teething or vaccinations. However, a rectal temperature of 100.4°F (38°C) or higher in a baby under three months should prompt an immediate call to your pediatrician.

Breastfeeding Myths and Truths

1. **Myth: Small Breasts Can't Produce Enough Milk**

   - **Truth**: Breast size doesn't affect milk production. Milk supply depends on demand, so frequent breastfeeding or pumping helps maintain an adequate supply.

2. **Myth: Formula-Fed Babies Are Less Healthy**

   - **Truth**: While breastfeeding has many benefits, formula is a safe and nutritious alternative for babies. A well-fed baby—regardless of feeding method—is a healthy baby.

3. **Myth: You Can't Breastfeed if You're Sick**

   - **Truth**: Most illnesses don't affect breastfeeding, and antibodies in your milk can help protect your baby from getting sick. Always check with your doctor if you're unsure.

Debunking Old Wives' Tales

1. **Myth: Hanging a Wedding Ring on a String Predicts Your Baby's Gender**

   - **Truth**: This is purely a fun superstition with no scientific basis.

2. **Myth: Babies Born with a Lot of Hair Cause Heartburn**

   - **Truth**: While there's limited evidence linking hormones responsible for heartburn to hair growth, this isn't a guaranteed correlation.

3. **Myth: Walking Barefoot Causes Colds**

   - **Truth**: Colds are caused by viruses, not cold feet. Keeping warm and comfortable is still important, especially for your baby.

How to Approach Myths

1. **Do Your Research**

   - Use reliable sources like medical professionals, reputable parenting websites, and updated books.

2. **Consult Your Pediatrician**

   - When in doubt, seek advice from your baby's doctor.

3. **Trust Your Instincts**

   - Every parent-child relationship is unique. Balance expert advice with what feels right for you and your baby.

By separating fact from fiction, you can approach pregnancy and parenthood with greater confidence and less stress.

Chapter 15: Building a Support System

Parenting is not a solo endeavor. Building a reliable support system can provide you with the emotional, physical, and logistical help you need during pregnancy, childbirth, and the early months of your baby's life.

Why a Support System Matters

1. **Emotional Support**

    - Pregnancy and early parenthood can bring a mix of joy, stress, and uncertainty. Having people to lean on can help you navigate these emotions.

2. **Practical Assistance**

    - From preparing meals to helping with household chores, a support system lightens your load so you can focus on your baby and yourself.

3. **Guidance and Advice**

    - Experienced parents in your circle can share tips and lessons learned. While their experiences may not mirror yours, their advice can be valuable.

Who to Include in Your Support System

1. **Your Partner**

   - **Role**: Provides emotional encouragement, helps with baby care, and shares household responsibilities.

   - **Tips for Involvement**:

     - Attend prenatal classes together.

     - Communicate openly about your needs and concerns.

     - Share baby duties, such as feeding or diaper changes.

2. **Family Members**

   - Grandparents, siblings, and other relatives can offer love, practical help, and childcare support.

   - Be clear about boundaries and the type of help you'd appreciate to ensure harmony.

3. **Friends**

   - Close friends can offer emotional support, companionship, and even a listening ear when you need to vent or celebrate small milestones.

4. **Healthcare Professionals**

   - Your doctor, midwife, or pediatrician can provide expert advice and reassurance.

   - Consider a lactation consultant or postpartum doula for specialized support.

5. Parenting Communities

- Join local or online parenting groups to connect with others experiencing similar challenges and joys.

- These groups often share resources, tips, and camaraderie.

How to Build Your Support Network

1. Communicate Your Needs

- Don't hesitate to ask for help, whether it's babysitting, meal prep, or just a conversation.

- Be specific about what you need to avoid misunderstandings.

2. Cultivate Relationships Early

- Strengthen connections with friends and family during pregnancy so they're ready to step in after your baby arrives.

3. Leverage Technology

- Use apps or group chats to coordinate schedules and stay in touch with your support network.

- Join online forums or social media groups tailored to pregnancy and parenting.

4. Plan for Emergencies

- Identify people you can rely on in urgent situations, like unexpected trips to the doctor.

- Keep important contact numbers easily accessible.

Maintaining Your Support System

1. **Express Gratitude**

   - A simple "thank you" or a small gesture of appreciation can go a long way in maintaining relationships.

2. **Reciprocate When Possible**

   - Offer support to others in your network when you're able, even if it's just lending a listening ear.

3. **Set Boundaries**

   - Politely decline advice or help that doesn't align with your parenting values or needs.

   - Prioritize your well-being and your baby's above all else.

When Professional Help Is Needed

1. **Postpartum Counseling**

   - If you're feeling overwhelmed, anxious, or depressed, a mental health professional can provide valuable tools and support.

2. **Specialized Services**

   - Consider hiring a lactation consultant, sleep coach, or childcare professional for specific challenges.

Remember, It Takes a Village

- Parenthood is a journey best undertaken with the love and support of others. By surrounding yourself with people who uplift and assist you, you'll create a nurturing environment for your baby and yourself.

Chapter 16: Reflection and Looking Ahead

As your pregnancy journey concludes and you transition into parenthood, it's important to take a moment to reflect on your experiences and set intentions for the future. This chapter focuses on celebrating your growth, embracing the unknown, and preparing for the next stage of your family's life.

Reflecting on Your Pregnancy Journey

1. **Celebrate Your Strength**

   - Pregnancy is a transformative experience that challenges you physically and emotionally. Acknowledge your resilience and adaptability.

2. **Cherish the Milestones**

   - Recall special moments: hearing your baby's heartbeat, feeling the first kicks, or sharing the news with loved ones.

3. **Learn from Challenges**

   - Reflect on any difficulties you faced, such as morning sickness, anxiety, or unexpected changes. Consider how these experiences have made you stronger.

4. **Gratitude for Support**

   - Take time to appreciate the people, professionals, and resources that supported you throughout your journey.

Looking Ahead: The Adventure of Parenthood

1. **Your New Identity as a Parent**

    - Parenthood brings new roles and responsibilities. Embrace the changes, but remember that it's okay to retain your individuality and pursue personal goals.

2. **Set Realistic Expectations**

    - Adjusting to life with a baby takes time. It's natural to face ups and downs as you find your rhythm.

    - Remember that there's no "perfect parent," only one who loves, learns, and grows.

3. **Embrace Flexibility**

    - Babies don't come with manuals, and parenting often requires quick thinking and adaptability. Trust your instincts and seek help when needed.

Creating a Vision for Your Family

1. **Prioritize Connection**

    - Foster a nurturing and supportive environment for your baby and your partner.

    - Dedicate time to family bonding, whether through daily routines or special outings.

2. **Set Goals Together**

    - Discuss long-term plans with your partner, such as career aspirations, financial goals, or future family plans.

3. **Build Traditions**

    - Start family traditions that reflect your values and create cherished memories.

Self-Care in Parenthood

1. **Continue Caring for Yourself**

    - Self-care doesn't end with pregnancy. Prioritize sleep, nutrition, and mental health as you navigate parenthood.

2. **Celebrate Small Wins**

    - Every successful diaper change, feeding, or milestone is a victory worth acknowledging.

3. **Stay Connected with Your Support Network**

    - Maintain relationships with friends, family, and other parents. Shared experiences can provide valuable support and perspective.

Documenting Your Journey

1. **Capture Memories**

   - Take photos, write in a journal, or create a scrapbook to preserve precious moments.

2. **Write Letters to Your Baby**

   - Share your thoughts, hopes, and dreams for your child in letters they can read later in life.

Final Words of Encouragement

Parenthood is a journey of discovery, growth, and love. While it can feel overwhelming at times, it's also filled with unparalleled joy and fulfillment. Trust in your ability to provide a safe, loving, and enriching environment for your child.

Remember, you are not alone. Lean on your partner, family, friends, and the wider parenting community as you navigate this incredible chapter of life.

Your story is just beginning, and the best is yet to come.

Conclusion

As your journey through pregnancy and the early stages of parenthood unfolds, remember that you are on a path filled with love, learning, and growth. Every challenge you face and every joy you experience will shape the kind of parent you become, and no two experiences are ever the same. It's okay to make mistakes, seek help, and adjust your approach as needed.

Take a deep breath and embrace the beautiful chaos of life with a baby. Cherish every moment, whether it's a sleepless night or a first smile. These fleeting moments will soon turn into precious memories that will last a lifetime.

Above all, know that you are doing an amazing job. Whether you're pregnant with your first child or welcoming a new sibling into the family, each day is a step toward creating a loving and nurturing environment for your growing family.

Thank you for taking this journey with me. I hope this book has provided you with the guidance, encouragement, and confidence you need as you embark on this exciting new chapter.

Acknowledgments

I would like to express my heartfelt gratitude to everyone who has been a part of this book.

First and foremost, to all the expectant and new parents who are navigating this beautiful and sometimes challenging journey, your experiences are the inspiration for this book. Thank you for trusting in the process and for sharing your stories.

To the healthcare professionals—doctors, nurses, midwives, and doulas—who provide unwavering support, guidance, and care to families every day. Your expertise and compassion are invaluable.

To my family and friends, thank you for your continuous love, encouragement, and support throughout the writing of this book. Your belief in me kept me motivated.

Lastly, to my partner, for your endless patience and understanding throughout this process, and for always being by my side.

This book would not have been possible without the collective support of all those who have offered their knowledge, love, and encouragement.